KT-150-753

About the CD

It is strongly recommended that you listen to the CD using high quality headphones or speakers. The minimum system requirements are:

Apple Macintosh
Any model using OS 7.5 or higher

Windows for PC
Pentium II processor or higher
Windows 98 or newer
4x times CD-ROM drive or faster
Sound card

Installation
1. Insert the CD-ROM and double-click on the CD icon on the desktop.

2. Double-click on the 'macstart' icon.

Installation
1. Insert the CD-ROM

2. The CD should start automatically.

3. If the CD does not start, Browse to your CD drive and Run

Getting started

1. To select the area you wish to learn about, click on the appropriate button.

2. Select a heart sound by clicking on it.

3. You now have a choice of either listening to the tutorial or using the interactive software yourself (the manipulator). We recommend that with each heart sound you listen to the tutorial first, in conjunction with the text for the tutorial as it appears in the book 🔊. Subsequently you can use the tutorial in the book to reproduce the sounds manually through the manipulator or experiment with the manipulator yourself.

4. In the manipulator you need to press **Stop** to stop the recording in order to manipulate it. Then press **Start** to continue.

5. When you have manipulated a part of the cardiac cycle and restarted the manipulator you will hear a change, which is reflected by a visual change in the phonocardiogram.

6. To return to the native recording press **Reset**.

Technical support
e-mail: cdrom@eslo.co.uk
Telephone: +44 (0) 20 7611 4202

Heart Sounds
Made Easy

Commissioning Editor: Laurence Hunter
Project Development Manager: Siân Jarman
Project Manager: Nancy Arnott
Designer: Erik Bigland
CD developer: Clive Marklew
Illustrator: Graeme Chambers

Heart Sounds Made Easy

E. M. Brown
Associate Specialist
Wessex Cardiothoracic Centre
Southampton General Hospital
Southampton, UK

W. Collis
Institute of Sound and Vibration Research
Southampton University
Southampton, UK

T. Leung
Institute of Sound and Vibration Research
Southampton University
Southampton, UK

A. P. Salmon
Consultant Paediatric Cardiologist
Wessex Cardiothoracic Centre
Southampton General Hospital
Southampton, UK

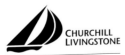

CHURCHILL
LIVINGSTONE

EDINBURGH LONDON NEW YORK OXFORD PHILADELPHIA ST LOUIS SYDNEY
TORONTO 2002

CHURCHILL LIVINGSTONE
An imprint of Elsevier Science Limited

First Published 2002
  Reprinted 2003

ISBN 0-443-07141-1

British Library Cataloguing in Publication Data
A catalogue record for this book is available from the British Library

Library of Congress Cataloging in Publication Data
A catalog record for this book is available from the Library of Congress

Note
Medical knowledge is constantly changing. As new information
becomes available, changes in treatment, procedures, equipment and the
use of drugs become necessary. The authors and the publishers have
taken care to ensure that the information given in this text is accurate
and up to date. However, readers are strongly advised to confirm that
the information, especially with regard to drug usage, complies with the
latest legislation and standards of practice.

ELSEVIER SCIENCE
your source for books,
journals and multimedia
in the health sciences

www.elsevierhealth.com

The
publisher's
policy is to use
**paper manufactured
from sustainable forests**

Typeset by IMH(Cartrif), Loanhead, Scotland
Printed in China
C/03

Preface

Cardiac auscultation is one of the most difficult skills to acquire and competence in this area is extremely variable. Until now teaching has been bedside with an expert describing the physical signs and the trainee nodding knowingly. The main skill acquired is the ability to appear knowledgeable while remaining mystified. This method of teaching does not allow the trainer or trainee to verify that they are appreciating the specific auscultatory features in the different parts of the cardiac cycle. We want to give you the opportunity to learn auscultation skills as if you have a consultant cardiologist present to teach you at your convenience. We have therefore written what we hope is a short and accessible book which takes you through the questions that we ask ourselves when we listen to heart sounds. This can be used alone or in conjunction with the CD of heart sounds recorded from actual patients.

The unique feature of the Heart Sounds Made Easy CD is that it is an interactive tool based on the latest digital audio technology. It allows the user to listen to a recording and either eliminate or enhance the different components until they are confident that they have correctly identified the sounds in all phases of the cardiac cycle. This is particularly important for the recognition of diastolic sounds which are the most difficult to appreciate. There is no better way to confirm the presence of such a murmur than to have the facility to reduce or increase its intensity. This software is now used routinely for teaching auscultation to students and junior doctors on the Wessex Cardiothoracic Unit in Southampton, where it has proved successful and popular. We hope that you will find it equally valuable as an educational aid.

Southampton	E.M.B.
2002	W.C.
	T.L.
	A.P.S.

Acknowledgements

First and foremost we wish to thank all the patients and their families for allowing us to record their heart sounds. We must also thank the staff and trustees of Wessex Heartbeat for all their support in developing the heart sound manipulator and providing the funds to help develop this technology and CD. We would like to express our particular gratitude to Alan Prince, who as chairman of Wessex Heartbeat Trustees maintained the momentum necessary for the completion of this project as well as all the audio-visual facilities. Thanks to Paul White, Antonello de Stefano and Alfredo Giani at the Institute of Sound and Vibration Research at Southampton University for their help in developing the CD software. Finally a very big thank you to Clive Marklew for all his work on producing a CD which satisfied all the different demands of the authors and publishers.

Contents

How to use the book and CD

The *Heart Sounds Made Easy* book and CD-rom can be used together or separately. Each chapter of the book corresponds to a region of the chest and the corresponding sounds. For each heart sound you should read the information in the relevant chapter to familiarize yourself with the anatomy, history, examination, and characteristics of a particular heart sound. You should then listen to the relevant tutorial on the CD-rom.

The CD is best listened to through high quality headphones or good quality speakers. Listening through headphones gives an experience closer to that of listening through a stethoscope than does using speakers. The PC version requires a Pentium class machine or better. On inserting the CD into your computer it should start automatically. If not, for the PC version choose My Computer, and double click on the CD drive. For the Macintosh version, insert the CD-ROM into the drive and double click on the **macstart** icon.

The initial screen allows you to choose the 1st Time Users button, which is an introduction to the aims of the CD. The credits button gives information on the organizations involved in producing the CD-rom and book.

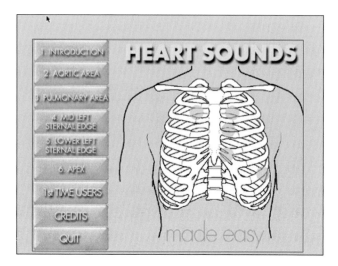

This screen also shows the contents, containing chapter headings that correspond with those in the book. Chose the area you are interested in and click on the button. You will then see a screen that shows a list of the heart sounds best heard in that area. This corresponds to the sounds discussed in that chapter of the book. Choose the heart sound you are interested in. You then have a choice of listening to a tutorial or using the interactive software yourself (the manipulator). The tutorial will give you an overview of the sounds and their main characteristics. During the tutorial the cursors are automatically manipulated and they do not flash. Note that the phonocardiogram is colour coded, with the colours corresponding to those on the cursors below. The tutorial does not allow you to hear the heart sounds at their best and should only be used as an initial guide. You must use the manipulator in order to hear the heart sounds clearly.

Once you have listened to the tutorial use the manipulator to reproduce the tutorial for yourself using the transcript that appears in the book. If you are using a PC a dialogue box saying 'Loading Manipulator' will appear. Click 'OK' and wait until the manipulator loads. (Note: on Windows 2000 the manipulator may appear as a blank screen. If this occurs you should minimize then remaximize the window. The manipulator will then appear.) If using a Macintosh there will be a brief pause while the manipulator loads.

On the manipulator you will notice that the cursors do flash in conjunction with the heart sounds. When you are using the manipulator, the cursor hitting systole coincides with S_1 and hitting diastole coincides with S_2. When you have manipulated a part of the cardiac cycle there is a change in the phonocardiogram to visually represent this change. You need to **Stop** the recording in order to manipulate it, and to return to the native recording press **Reset**.

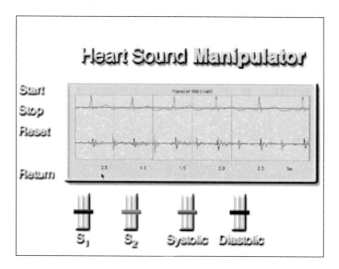

Use the manipulator to reproduce the tutorial as many times as you need to in order to fully appreciate the subtleties of the sounds you are listening to. You can then use the manipulator to vary the components of the heart sounds in any way you wish. Doing this will also help you to identify the sounds both individually and in combination.

When you have finished press **Return**. On a PC you will return to the screen for the heart sound you have been listening to. Click **Back** or **Contents** to navigate to another sound or area. On the Macintosh you will be returned to the main contents screen. From here you can return to the same area or chose a different one.

When you have finished press **Stop** and **Back** to return to the previous screen. To exit the CD keep pressing **Back** until you reach a screen with **Quit**.

Chapter 1

Introduction

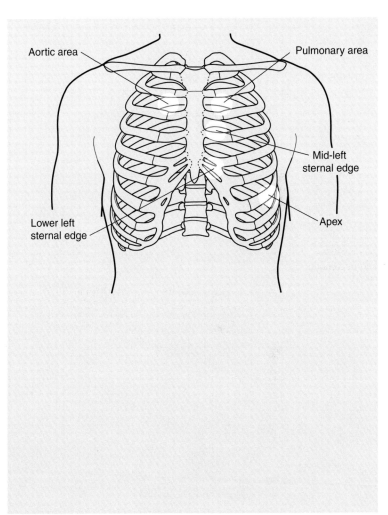

This book focuses on auscultation skills in the assessment of the cardiovascular system; however, as in all areas of clinical medicine, the history and remainder of the clinical examination are equally important, and it is vital to be systematic and consistent in your approach to diagnosis. The clinician must have a routine that ensures that no part of the history or clinical examination is missed. It is also important to remember that a patient can have severe cardiovascular disease in the absence of any abnormal physical signs and grossly abnormal physical signs may be detected in an asymptomatic patient.

Stethoscope

A high quality stethoscope is an important investment and most can last a lifetime. The authors feel that an adult cardiological stethoscope is suitable for *all* ages and that these have better acoustic features than the smaller paediatric and neonatal stethoscopes. The bell is designed to pick up lower frequency sounds, such as the diastolic murmur of mitral stenosis, and the diaphragm picks up most other sounds. The longer the tube, the more likely it is for the sound to be dissipated: the standard length is recommended (approximately 50 cm). Remember that the best stethoscope cannot compete with background noise or an uncooperative patient!

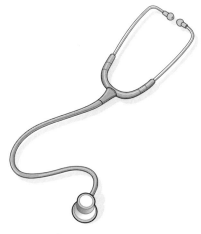

Fig. 1.1   *Stethoscope*

History

Although there are a large number of cardiovascular diseases, there are only a handful of possible symptoms. Exertional chest pain is most frequently associated with coronary artery disease, but hypertrophic cardiomyopathy and severe outflow tract obstruction may result in cardiac pain. Cardiac disease also frequently produces breathlessness, initially on exertion but in severe disease ultimately at rest. A history of orthopnoea or paroxysmal nocturnal dyspnoea are highly suggestive of cardiac as opposed to respiratory disease. Palpitations are a frequent symptom in the population and usually only represent an awareness of normal sinus tachycardia; however, palpitations related to arrhythmias may be the presenting feature of many different cardiac conditions. Syncope is most commonly vasovagal in origin but this is a diagnosis of exclusion, as syncope may reflect life-threatening cardiac disease. Swelling of the ankles due to dependent oedema is frequently not associated with cardiac disease but is a feature of congestive cardiac failure.

No history is complete without an assessment of cardiovascular risk: this includes family history, smoking, hypertension, diabetes and lipid status.

General physical examination

General examination will include assessment of the height and weight of the patient. Obesity is an important risk factor added stress in patients with cardiovascular disease. Tall thin stature may be part of the Marfan syndrome. Xanthelasmas are an important sign of raised serum cholesterol. The presence of distal and central cyanosis should be sought, along with finger clubbing. The presence of oedema, initially of the legs but in severe heart failure eventually generalized, including ascites and pleural effusions, should be specifically sought.

Structural heart disease is more common in patients with other congenital abnormalities than in the general population; it is therefore important to look carefully for any dysmorphic features in the face, or abnormalities in other systems, particularly in the skeletal or gastrointestinal system.

As with all physical examination, it is important to have the patient fully undressed. When examining children, however, it is sometimes the case that trying to get them undressed may upset them so much that it is impossible to listen to them and compromise is therefore necessary.

Cardiovascular examination

Arterial pulsation/blood pressure

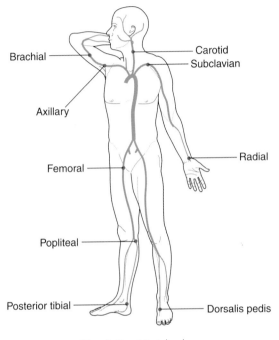

Fig. 1.2 *Arterial pulses*

The radial pulse is initially assessed for rate and rhythm. The character and volume are classically assessed at the carotid pulse, but, particularly in children, this may be distressing and the brachial pulse may be used. All the pulses should be palpated and the volume compared with the other side (not simultaneously in the case of the carotid pulse). The difference between the systolic and diastolic blood pressure measured with a sphygmomanometer gives an important objective measure of pulse pressure.

Venous pulsation

The central venous pulse is assessed with the patient lying comfortably at 45° and the height is described as centimetres above the clavicle. In normal patients the jugular venous pulse is not visible. It may be very difficult to assess, particularly in obese patients. A raised jugular venous pressure is an important sign of cardiac failure, or obstruction to the superior vena cava, in which case pulsation is lost.

Inspection of the chest

The chest should be inspected for signs of deformity, visible pulsation, enlarged veins and scars from previous surgery. In thin individuals the apex beat may be visible.

Palpation of the chest

The chest is palpated to determine the position of the cardiac apex, which is the lowest and outermost point where the cardiac pulsation is felt. The patient must be lying or sitting straight. In healthy individuals it will be in the mid-clavicular line, in the 5th intercostal space on the left. The position of the apex may be affected by the heart being displaced in the chest due to spine and rib deformities or lung disease, as well as cardiac disease. If the apex is difficult to define, do not forget to palpate on the right side of the chest for dextrocardia. The quality of the apex beat should be assessed but this is affected by subcutaneous fat. The apex should also be felt to check for thrills. The chest should then be palpated using the flat of the hand on the left and right of the sternum to feel for a right ventricular heave (*left of sternum*) and thrills on either side. The suprasternal notch is palpated to check for an aortic thrill.

Percussion of the chest

The cardiac dullness may be percussed but in practice this is not routinely done. Percussion of the chest is more useful to confirm liver size, and if significant pleural effusions are present.

Auscultation

Remember
- Heart sounds
- Added sounds
- Murmurs

Heart sounds

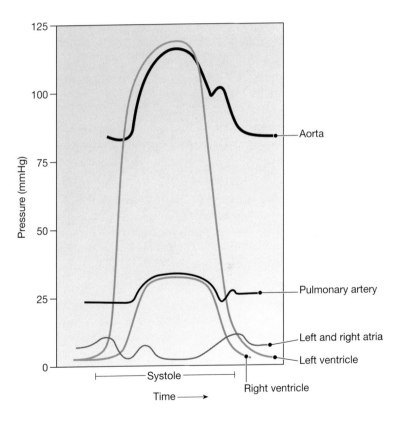

Fig. 1.3 *The cardiac cycle*

First heart sound S_1
The first heart sound is caused by the mitral and tricuspid valves closing at the beginning of systole. The mitral valve closes before the tricuspid valve, although it is not usually possible to appreciate the dual nature of the sound.

Second heart sound S_2
The second sound is caused by the closure of the aortic and then pulmonary valves. Because the delay is greater than in the first heart sound this usually can be heard. Normal splitting becomes wider with inspiration and narrower with expiration.

Added sounds
S_3 and S_4
The third and fourth heart sounds are low frequency sounds which occur in diastole. The third heart sound occurs in early diastole at the time of maximum ventricular filling. It may be heard in young fit adults and during pregnancy. The fourth heart sound occurs at the time of atrial contraction and is therefore only present if the patient is in sinus rhythm. Both these sounds are best heard with the bell of the stethoscope and with the patient turned slightly onto the left side.

Clicks and snaps
The opening of a normal heart valve is silent. Ejection clicks arise from an abnormal aortic or pulmonary valve as it opens, and occur early in systole. They may be mistaken for splitting of the first heart sound. An opening snap arises from an abnormal mitral or tricuspid valve and therefore is heard in diastole. Note that as the valve becomes more severely affected and the movement is decreased the click or snap will disappear.

Knock and rub
In constrictive pericarditis there may be a loud, low frequency diastolic noise known as a knock. A pericardial rub is a high frequency noise, loudest in systole, but often present in diastole as well. A rub may vary from hour to hour, and if a significant effusion develops the rub will disappear.

Murmurs
As with the whole cardiovascular examination it is important to have a systematic approach to describing a murmur. The timing of a murmur (systolic or diastolic) may be difficult, particularly if the patient is tachycardic. Systole

may be timed by feeling the carotid pulse in the neck. Murmurs are systolic, diastolic, systolic and diastolic or continuous. The timing of murmurs is discussed in the relevant chapters.

Murmurs may be low pitched, such as mitral stenosis, or high pitched, such as small ventricular septal defects (VSDs). Murmurs vary in intensity but it is important to note that loud murmurs do not necessarily indicate severe disease. For example, small VSDs may give loud murmurs, whereas large ones may produce no murmur. Systolic murmurs are traditionally graded out of 6, with a 1/6 murmur being quiet and a 6/6 being very loud. Diastolic murmurs are graded out of four.

Table 1.1   Grading of systolic murmurs

Grade	Thrill	Murmur
1/6	Absent	Very quiet
2/6	Absent	Quiet
3/6	Absent	Easily audible
4/6	Present	Loud
5/6	Present	Audible with stethoscope half off chest
6/6	Present	Audible without stethoscope

It is also important to determine whether the murmur changes during respiration. Typically, murmurs arising from the right heart are accentuated on inspiration.

We have arranged this book by the position where the murmur is loudest. This is because we feel that we rely particularly on this feature to identify a murmur. It is also important to determine where else a murmur is heard, or the *radiation,* as this also gives important information on the source of the murmur.

Investigations

Electrocardiogram and chest radiograph

The electrocardiogram (ECG) and chest X-ray (CXR) give important information that may help to confirm a diagnosis or help to assess severity. We have therefore included a short note on possible ECG and CXR features, although detailed descriptions of the abnormalities are beyond the scope of this book.

Echocardiogram, cardiac catheterization and magnetic resonance imaging

Full assessment of cardiac pathology increasingly includes the use of echocardiography, and this service is being offered in many district general hospitals, although cardiac catheterization and cardiac magnetic resonance imaging remain the province of specialist centres. It is, however, vital to understand that an accurate echocardiographic assessment depends upon accurate assessment of the clinical findings.

> **Learning point**
> • You only find what you look for.

❿ 1.1 Normal heart sounds

Remember that the recognition of abnormal heart sounds depends on the ability to appreciate, with certainty, the normal heart sounds.

Start

Listen to the recording. Focus on S_1 while watching the systolic diastolic cursor (SDC) and note that S_1 coincides with the SDC landing on systole. When confident of timing of S_1, focus on S_2: note that S_2 coincides with the SDC landing on diastole.

Stop

Minimize S_1

Start

Note the normal phonocardiogram without an S_1.

Stop

Reset

Minimize S_2

Note the normal phonocardiogram without an S_2.

Stop

Reset

Start

Listen again to the native recording. Stop the recording and listen after increasing S_1 and S_2 to maximum if you wish.

1.2 Third heart sound

Start

Listen to the recording. Focus on S_1 while watching the SDC and note that S_1 coincides with the SDC landing on systole. When confident of the timing of S_1 focus on S_2. Note that S_2 coincides with the SDC landing on diastole. Note the third heart sound in diastole.

Stop

Minimize Diastole

Start

The third heart sound has now been eliminated.

Stop

Reset

Start

Listen again to the native recording. It is easy to hear why this has been likened to a galloping horse.

Stop

Repeat until you are confident that you can identify the third heart sound in diastole.

Chapter 2

Aortic area
(upper right sternal edge)

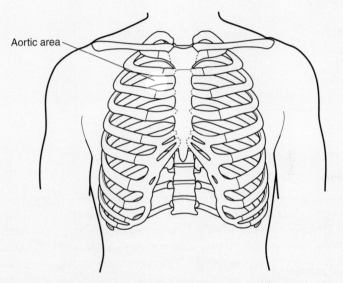

Aortic area

The aortic area is in the second right intercostal space

The murmurs best heard in this region are:
- Aortic stenosis
- Venous hum

Aortic stenosis

Anatomy

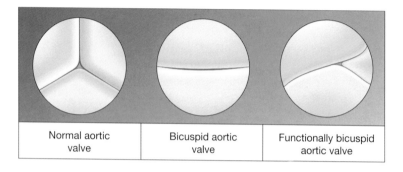

| Normal aortic valve | Bicuspid aortic valve | Functionally bicuspid aortic valve |

Fig. 2.1 *Aortic valve*

The aortic valve usually has three equal sized cusps. The valve may be narrowed due to fusion between these cusps, or due to a valve with only two or even one cusp. Typically, even in a trileaflet valve, the cusps are not of equal size. In congenital aortic stenosis, the valve annulus may also be small, and this is particularly true when the mitral valve is abnormal, or coarctation is also present (the Shone syndrome).

The aortic valve may also be narrowed due to thickening and myxomatous change in the valve. Don't forget that aortic regurgitation may co-exist in any patient with aortic stenosis (see Chapter 4, p. 48).

History

Aortic stenosis will usually be asymptomatic and detected because of the presence of a murmur, although patients may have angina, syncope on exercise, and rarely present with sudden death on exertion. The left ventricle will eventually fail and then the patient will develop breathlessness.

In neonates, critical aortic stenosis presents as a collapsed child with absent or very feeble pulses, respiratory distress and an enlarged liver.

Examination

In mild aortic stenosis, the general examination will be normal. In moderate to severe disease, the pulses may be of small volume and the pulse pressure narrow on blood pressure measurement. There may be a thrill in the suprasternal notch, or in more severe disease in the aortic area. The apex beat may be tapping in quality.

As already described, neonates may present collapsed with very poor pulses.

Heart sounds	S_1 normal
	S_2 normal or soft
Added sounds	Ejection click after S_1, loudest at the apex
Murmurs	Ejection systolic murmur in the aortic area radiating into the neck

ECG

In mild stenosis this will be normal. With increasing severity left ventricular hypertrophy and then strain will develop.

CXR

This may well be normal, although post-stenotic dilatation of the ascending aorta may be seen and does not relate to severity. Left ventricular hypertrophy may be visible in moderate to severe hypertrophy, and if the left ventricle fails, signs of raised left ventricular filling pressures and pulmonary oedema will be seen.

Notes

The severity of aortic stenosis may progress throughout life. At the mildest end of the spectrum there may be only an ejection click from a bicuspid valve, not associated with stenosis or regurgitation. In patients with stenosis an ejection systolic murmur is heard, which is louder in more severe disease until the stenosis becomes severe and the cardiac output is compromised. The onset of left ventricular failure will further contribute to a reduction in the intensity of the murmur.

Learning points
- The murmur of aortic stenosis is loudest in the aortic area but the click is loudest at the apex.
- An abnormal aortic valve may be associated with coarctation of the aorta.
- In very severe aortic stenosis, particularly when left ventricular failure supervenes, the murmur may be soft.

2.1 Aortic stenosis—valvar (click)

Start

There is only a very soft systolic murmur and the main feature of this recording is an ejection click. The click is best heard at the apex, where this recording was made. The click occurs almost immediately after S_1 and is very difficult to separate from it. Inexperienced auscultators often describe S_1 as being 'split', which is indeed what it sounds like. We will now manipulate the intensity of the click to try to help you appreciate it better.

Stop

Maximize Click

Start

You have increased the intensity of the click and it should be clearer to you. Think of it as sounding like splitting of S_1. Watch the SDC and time the heart sounds while trying to appreciate the click.

Stop

Minimize Click

Maximize S_1

Start

Listen to the heart sounds and note the click has gone and S_1 sounds single, loud and discrete.

Stop

Maximise Click

Minimise S_1

Start

Listen carefully: S_1 has gone and only the click is present (which sounds remarkably like S_1).

Stop

Leave Click on maximum

Maximize S$_1$

Start

Both S$_1$ and click are now accentuated. The 'double' sound is apparent. Listen while watching the SDC.

Stop

Reset

Start

Listen to the native recording and watch the SDC. Confirm that you appreciate the click and its close relationship to S$_1$.

2.2 Aortic stenosis (murmur)

Start

Listen to the recording. This murmur was recorded in the aortic area where the murmur of aortic stenosis is loudest and the click is often inaudible. You will recall that the click is best heard at the apex. Note the soft first heart sound and the ejection systolic murmur which is clearly followed by S_2.

Stop

Minimize Systole

Start

Only S_1 and S_2 are now audible. Time these sounds with the SDC. S_1 coincides with Systole and S_2 with Diastole.

Stop

Maximize Systole

Start

Appreciate the loud systolic murmur.

Stop

Reset

Start

Listen finally to the native recording.

Summary		
• Where is the murmur loudest?	→	Aortic area
• When does the murmur occur?	→	Systole
• What else could it be?	→	Still's murmur sometimes audible here but usually at the lower left sternal edge
• What makes it valvar aortic stenosis?	→	Quality of murmur, radiation into neck, click or thrill if present

Venous hum

Anatomy

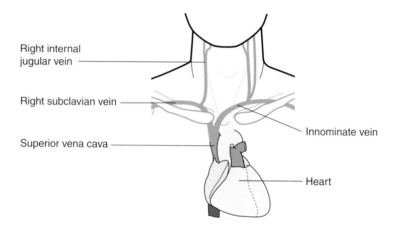

Fig. 2.2 *Great veins in the neck*

A venous hum is a common innocent murmur of childhood and by definition the cardiac anatomy is normal. The continuous noise originates from the great veins in the neck.

History

The patient will be asymptomatic. Venous hums are commonest from age 12 months to 6 years and so these murmurs are often detected on routine screening medical examinations. They may also be present in fit young adults, but also occur with a hyperdynamic circulation, such as in pregnancy, thyrotoxicosis or anaemia.

Examination

General examination will be normal.

Heart sounds	S_1 normal
	S_2 normal
Added sounds	Nil
Murmurs	A continuous murmur, maximum above the clavicles but often audible in the aortic and pulmonary areas

ECG

This will be normal.

CXR

This will be normal.

Notes

Venous hums are low pitched continuous murmurs which are actually loudest above the clavicle, but are often heard below the clavicle, and are usually louder on the right than the left. They are accentuated by asking the subject to look over his or her shoulder and upwards, and are loudest when sitting and disappear when lying flat. They may be abolished by getting the subject to look in front and slightly downwards, or more reliably by pressure on the jugular vein, just lateral to the sternocleidomastoid muscle.

Learning point
- A venous hum is a common innocent murmur in childhood.

2.3 Venous hum

Start

Listen to the recording. There is a soft continuous murmur. The most difficult part of the murmur to appreciate is the diastolic component. Most trainees initially interpret this as a systolic murmur. We will now demonstrate its presence throughout the cardiac cycle. Listen carefully. The murmur is audible throughout systole and diastole. Watch the SDC. The second heart sound in this example is loud. Try to appreciate the murmur as it travels *through* S_2.

Stop

Minimize Diastole

Start

You will now hear only the systolic component of this murmur and S_2 is the clearly defined end point. Watch the SDC while listening carefully and you will hear the whole of diastole is now silent—there is silence after the second heart sound.

Stop

Maximize Diastole

Start

The diastolic component is louder than before. Listen until you are confident of its presence.

Stop

Minimize Systole (leaving Diastole maximized)

Start

The murmur is purely diastolic. In this example you can still hear S_2, which now coincides with the beginning of the diastolic murmur (S_2 coincides with the SDC hitting diastole).

Stop

Reset

Start

Listen to the native murmur and be sure you appreciate its quality and timing. Play with the heart sounds manipulator and restart as often as necessary. Become confident of the timing of diastole!

Summary	
• Where is the murmur loudest?	➔ Above the clavicle
• When does the murmur occur?	➔ Throughout systole and diastole
• What else could it be?	➔ A patent ductus arteriosus if loudest on the left
• What makes it a venous hum?	➔ Variability with posture and pressure in the neck

Chapter 3

Pulmonary area
(upper left sternal edge)

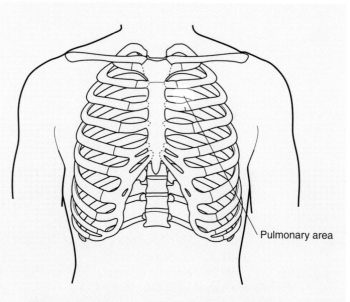

Pulmonary area

The pulmonary area is in the second left intercostal space

The auscultatory abnormalities best heard in this region are:
- Atrial septal defect
- Pulmonary stenosis
- Innocent pulmonary flow
- Patent ductus arteriosus
- Loud second heart sound

Atrial septal defect

Anatomy

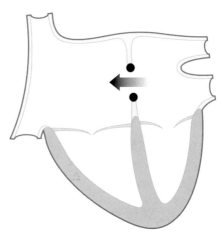

Fig. 3.1 *Atrial septal defect*

An atrial septal defect (ASD) is a hole in the atrial septum. Since the right atrial pressure is, for most of the time, lower than the left atrial pressure, this allows blood to flow from left atrium to right atrium. This leads to:

1. increase in size (dilatation) of the right atrium and ventricle
2. increased blood flow to the lungs.

At times, such as after straining (for example during childbirth), the right atrial pressure exceeds the left atrial pressure, which causes the flow to be right to left across the ASD.

Most commonly the hole is in the region of the normal fetal structure, the fossa ovalis (secundum ASD). The hole may be at the atrioventricular valve junction and is then associated with abnormal atrioventricular valves and mitral regurgitation (primum ASD, partial/incomplete atrioventricular septal defect.) The hole may be at the junction of the superior vena cava or inferior vena cava with the right atrium, and is then associated with partial anomalous pulmonary venous drainage. *However, the signs and symptoms in each case are identical.*

History

ASDs are often asymptomatic until complications arise in adulthood; however, they may be associated with chestiness and failure to thrive in childhood.

Complications arise from the physiological changes detailed above and are thus:

1. atrial or ventricular arrhythmias
2. frequent chest infections and eventually pulmonary hypertension due to increased pulmonary blood flow
3. stroke due to paradoxical embolism.

Examination

As always, look for signs of any recognizable syndrome. Down syndrome is particularly associated with ostium primum ASDs. Feel for right ventricular heave (from dilated right heart or pulmonary hypertension) and a palpable second heart sound (only in pulmonary hypertension.)

Heart sounds	S_1 normal
	S_2 widely split
Added sounds	Nil
Murmurs	Systole: ejection systolic murmur, often transmitted to the back.
	Diastole: usually silent or soft tricuspid flow murmur.

ECG

The ECG may be normal. It may show a rightward axis, prolonged PR interval and incomplete right bundle branch block. Ostium primum defects and some sinus venosus defects are associated with a superior axis. If there is pulmonary hypertension then voltage criteria for right ventricular hypertrophy may be satisfied.

CXR

This shows a large heart, particularly the right atrium, right ventricle and central pulmonary arteries. The lung fields will appear plethoric, although if pulmonary hypertension develops there will be peripheral pruning of the vessels.

Notes

ASDs vary in size from only a few millimetres to almost complete absence of the septum. There is therefore a range of haemodynamics, which is mirrored by the auscultatory findings. Classical teaching describes *wide fixed splitting* and indeed this is usually the case in *large* defects. In smaller defects, the second sound may be more narrowly split and somewhat variable, and sometimes difficult to differentiate from normal splitting. With the establishment of pulmonary hypertension the pulmonary component will become accentuated and the splitting reduced. The intensity of the pulmonary ejection murmur varies and, somewhat surprisingly, does not always correlate with defect size; however, the presence of a tricuspid diastolic murmur does suggest heavy flow through a large defect.

> **Learning points**
> - The classic signs of an ASD are not found if pulmonary hypertension supervenes.
> - Wide fixed splitting occurs in large defects.
> - Smaller ASDs may be associated with narrower splitting, which may be somewhat variable.

3.1 Atrial septal defect

Start

Listen to the recording. This is one of the most difficult diagnoses to make in cardiology. The murmur is soft and systolic and the main clue to the underlying aetiology is the wide fixed splitting of S_2. Listen carefully: splitting of the second sound, even when it is wide, is subtle. Note that S_2 occurs as the SDC hits diastole. Splitting may be likened to tapping the middle (first) and index (second) fingers of your right hand *almost* simultaneously onto a wooden table.

Stop

Minimize Systole

Start

You have eliminated the systolic murmur and you can now focus your attention onto S_2. Try to appreciate the splitting and don't worry, it is not that obvious.

Stop

Maximize the S_2 Split

Start

Listen carefully and focus on S_2. The systolic murmur is quiet and we have widened the splitting, making it easier to appreciate. Listen until you feel you can appreciate the splitting.

Stop

Minimize S_2 Splitting

Start

Listen carefully. The second sound remains somewhat split, but less than before.

Stop

Reset

Start

Listen to the native recording and be sure you appreciate the splitting of S_2 as well as the soft systolic murmur. Play with the heart sounds manipulator, increasing and decreasing the intensity of the murmur and increasing and decreasing the split of S_2 until you are confident of the heart sounds audible in a patient with an ASD. Become confident in appreciating a split S_2.

Summary	
• Where is the murmur loudest?	→ Pulmonary area
• When does the murmur occur?	→ Mid systole
• What else could it be?	→ Valvar pulmonary stenosis or innocent pulmonary flow murmur
• What makes it an ASD?	→ Presence of wide splitting of second sound

Valvar pulmonary stenosis

Anatomy

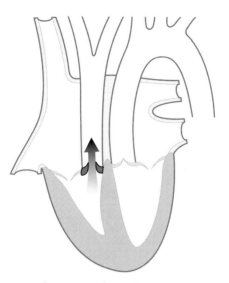

Fig. 3.2   *Valvar pulmonary stenosis*

Valvar pulmonary stenosis is narrowing at the level of the pulmonary valve. It may be due to fusion of the commissures of a bicuspid or tricuspid valve, or to a thickened myxomatous valve with limited movement. A very thickened dysplastic valve is more common in pulmonary stenosis associated with a syndrome (such as Noonan syndrome). The narrow valve leads to turbulent blood flow. The right ventricular pressure rises with increasing severity of stenosis in order to maintain blood flow to the lungs. As the stenosis becomes more severe, however, the right ventricle will be unable to overcome the obstruction and will fail.

History

Mild pulmonary stenosis is asymptomatic. It is detected because of the presence of a typical murmur, which is louder at times of high cardiac output, such as in a febrile illness or during pregnancy. Gradients across the pulmonary valve of less than 40 mmHg are unlikely to progress.

Moderate to severe pulmonary stenosis may also be asymptomatic, but may present with breathlessness and fatigue, particularly on exercise, due to the inability of the right ventricle to increase its output in the face of the limiting obstruction.

In the neonatal period, pulmonary stenosis may be critical, in which the cardiac output cannot be accommodated by the right heart. This may be associated with an anatomically small right ventricle. The baby will be well while the ductus arteriosus is patent, and if the foramen ovale allows right to left shunting of blood to bypass the right ventricle, but will become severely unwell when the duct shuts.

Examination

As always, look for signs of any recognizable syndrome. Noonan syndrome is particularly associated with pulmonary stenosis. General examination will usually be otherwise normal, although in severe pulmonary stenosis with right ventricular failure there may be a raised jugular venous pressure, ankle oedema and hepatomegaly. In critical pulmonary stenosis the baby will appear cyanosed and may be breathless and have a poor systemic cardiac output. In severe pulmonary stenosis there may be a right ventricular heave and a thrill palpable in the pulmonary area.

Heart sounds	S_1 normal
	S_2 normal
Added sounds	Systolic ejection click after first heart sound
Murmurs	Systole: ejection systolic murmur radiating through to back
	Diastole: usually nil

ECG

This will be normal in mild to moderate pulmonary stenosis, but will show right ventricular hypertrophy with right ventricular strain in severe cases. In Noonan syndrome there may be a superior axis. In neonates with critical pulmonary stenosis and a small right ventricle there may be an inappropriate lack of right ventricular forces present on the neonatal ECG.

CXR

This will usually be normal, although the main pulmonary artery may be prominent due to post-stenotic dilatation, which is not an indication of severity. In more severe pulmonary stenosis there will be right ventricular hypertrophy with an upturned cardiac apex, and cardiomegaly once the right ventricle has failed. In the neonate with critical pulmonary stenosis there will be pulmonary oligaemia, although the cardiac contour may be quite normal.

Notes

There may be an audible valve click. With increasing severity the click moves closer towards the first heart sound, so in very severe stenosis the click may become inaudible. There will be a systolic murmur that radiates through to the back. With increasing severity the murmur will become louder and may become associated with a thrill; however, with even more severe disease as the ventricle fails the murmur will become quieter again.

> **Learning point**
> - Valvar pulmonary stenosis may be part of complex congenital heart disease.

3.2 Pulmonary stenosis (valvar)

Start

Listen to the recording. This murmur was recorded in the pulmonary area. There is an ejection click just after S_1 and this is followed immediately by an ejection systolic murmur. We shall now manipulate the heart sounds.

Stop

Minimize Systole

Start

You have eliminated the systolic murmur and you can focus on the heart sounds. S_1 coincides with the SDC hitting systole. Immediately after S_1 is an ejection click. It is discrete and crisp and it is often mistaken for S_1 itself.

Stop

Minimize S_1

Start

Listen and note that most of the time there is no S_1, and the click is the first sound.

Stop

Maximize S_1

Start

Note S_1 immediately followed by the click.

Stop

Reset

Start

Listen to the native murmur and confirm in order S_1, ejection click, ejection systolic murmur and S_2. Use this case to learn to separate the click from S_1.

Summary	
• Where is the murmur loudest?	→ Pulmonary area
• When does the murmur occur?	→ Mid systole
• What else could it be?	→ ASD or innocent pulmonary flow murmur
• What makes it valvar pulmonary stenosis?	→ Presence of systolic click with variable splitting of second sound

Innocent pulmonary flow murmur

Anatomy

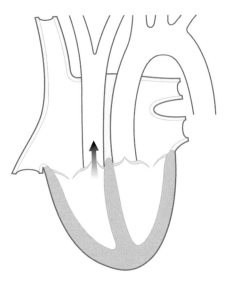

Fig. 3.3 *Innocent pulmonary flow murmur*

By definition the cardiac anatomy is normal in any innocent murmur. Pulmonary flow murmurs are, however, thought to arise from the right ventricular outflow tract.

History

These patients have structurally and functionally normal hearts, and therefore cannot have any cardiac symptoms. Innocent murmurs are very common in childhood and therefore by chance some children with symptoms such as chest pain, which are actually non-cardiac in origin, will have co-existing innocent murmurs.

Examination

The cardiovascular examination will be normal apart from the murmur. The presence of dysmorphic features makes structural heart disease more likely, but since innocent murmurs are common in childhood, there will by chance be some of these patients who have innocent murmurs.

Heart sounds	S_1 normal
	S_2 normal
Added sounds	Nil
Murmurs	Systole: Ejection systolic murmur
	Diastole: Nil

ECG

This will be normal.

CXR

This will be normal.

Notes

Innocent pulmonary flow murmurs are common, particularly in childhood, but also in young adults, especially in hyperdynamic states such as pregnancy. They do not radiate to the back.

Learning point
- The distinction between an innocent pulmonary flow murmur and an ASD depends upon assessment of the splitting of the second heart sound and may be very difficult.

◑ 3.3 Innocent pulmonary flow murmur

Start

Listen to the recording. This murmur has been recorded in the pulmonary area. Watch the SDC and note that the murmur coincides with it hitting systole and is very soft (1/6 in intensity). Try to appreciate S_1 and S_2, which are clearly and discretely audible. The main diagnostic feature of this murmur is that it is soft and does not radiate. We shall now manipulate the heart sounds.

Stop

Maximize Systole

Start

You have maximized this murmur and, if you could not hear it before, it should be more apparent now. Watch the SDC and time the two heart sounds.

Stop

Minimize Systole

Start

Listen and note the absence of the systolic murmur. In case you still have problems we will now maximize and minimize the murmur again to help you to appreciate it.

Stop

Maximize Systole

Start

Listen and appreciate the 'absence of nothing' in systole.

Stop

Minimize Systole

Start

Listen again to the silence in systole.

Stop

Reset

Start

Listen to the native murmur and be sure you can appreciate the soft systolic murmur.

Summary		
• Where is the murmur loudest?	→	Pulmonary area
• When does the murmur occur?	→	Mid systole
• What else could it be?	→	ASD or valvar pulmonary stenosis
• What makes it innocent pulmonary flow murmur?	→	Normal second sound and lack of radiation of murmur

Patent ductus arteriosus

Anatomy

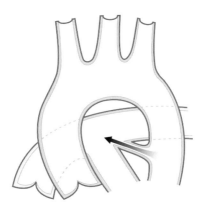

Fig. 3.4   *Patent ductus arteriosus*

The ductus arteriosus is a normal fetal structure that connects the main pulmonary artery with the descending aorta. It may remain patent after birth, particularly in babies born prematurely, sick newborns from any cause, and in the presence of structural heart disease. There is also a familial form of patent ductus arteriosus (PDA).

History

Large ducts may be associated with failure to thrive, and breathlessness or chestiness in childhood. Irreversible pulmonary hypertension may occur.

Examination

In large ducts the pulses will be full volume, with a wide pulse pressure (difference between systolic and diastolic blood pressure). The cardiac impulse will be active and the apex beat may be displaced towards the axilla due to enlargement of the left ventricle. The liver may be enlarged and there may be breathlessness, particularly in young babies. On auscultation there will be a continuous murmur audible throughout systole and into diastole. Note that continuous murmurs extend through the second sound but are not necessarily present throughout the whole cardiac cycle. The patent ductus murmur is loudest under the left clavicle, but may be audible throughout the precordium and posteriorly on the left. In large ducts there may be a mitral diastolic flow murmur audible at the apex.

Heart sounds	S_1 normal
	S_2 normal
Added sounds	Nil
Murmurs	Systole: continuous murmur, extending through second heart sound
	Diastole: continuous murmur, although may be quiet in late diastole

ECG

This will be normal in the presence of a small duct. Large ducts with large left to right shunts may show left ventricular volume overload with left ventricular hypertrophy on voltage criteria or generous biventricular voltages. If pulmonary hypertension develops there will be right ventricular hypertrophy, with right ventricular strain as the severity increases.

CXR

This will also be normal in small ducts. In the presence of a larger duct, the heart will enlarge (mainly the left ventricular contour) with pulmonary plethora and an enlarged pulmonary artery. With pulmonary hypertension, there will be an enlarged heart (mainly the right ventricle) with large central pulmonary arteries but peripheral pruning.

Notes

In large ducts there may be signs of 'heart failure', with hepatomegaly, failure to thrive and breathlessness. A wide pulse pressure, active precordium and mitral flow murmur are also signs of a large left to right shunt. If pulmonary hypertension supervenes, the continuous murmur will become quieter and shorter, and the second sound louder. With severe pulmonary hypertension, there will be a right ventricular heave, a loud and palpable second heart sound and pulmonary regurgitation may develop. Rarely, with reversal of the shunt through the duct there may be differential cyanosis and clubbing affecting the toes but not the fingers.

> **Learning point**
> • The murmur of a PDA may be mistaken for a venous hum.

3.4 Patent ductus arteriosus

Start

Listen to the recording. There is a continuous murmur which is described as machinery and is typical of a PDA. The murmur is loudest in the left infraclavicular region, where this recording was made. Time the murmur with the SDC. The systolic component is well appreciated. Try to appreciate the 'absence of nothing' in diastole, keeping focused on the SDC. We will now eliminate the diastolic component and attempt to hear the difference.

Stop

Minimize Diastole

Start

S_1 and S_2 are quite soft. Listen to the systolic murmur for a few cycles and note that there is 'nothing' after S_2 (during diastole). Watch the SDC while listening. Get the timing of each part of the cardiac cycle. Become familiar with the period of 'nothing' during diastole. We will now reintroduce the diastolic component at maximum intensity.

Stop

Maximize Diastole

Start

Watch the SDC. Note the systolic murmur. Note now the 'absence of nothing' when the SDC hits diastole. This is the diastolic component of the PDA murmur and the systolic and diastolic components run into each other, i.e. the murmur is continuous. Listen carefully for as long as it takes to appreciate fully this part of the murmur. If you are still having difficulty differentiating the systolic component from the diastolic then move on to the next stage.

Stop

Minimize Systole

Start

Note that there is now no systolic murmur. Watch the SDC and note that the murmur is purely diastolic with all the features described above.

Stop

Maximize Systole

Start

Both the systolic and diastolic components are set at maximum intensity. Listen until you are confident that you are clearly separating the two components.

Stop

Reset

Start

Listen finally to the native murmur and again time with the SDC. You should now be able to appreciate that the murmur runs through systole and diastole.

Summary	
• Where is the murmur loudest?	➔ Upper left sternal edge, under the clavicle
• When does the murmur occur?	➔ Throughout systole into diastole
• What else could it be?	➔ A venous hum is continuous but low pitched, louder in the neck and altered by pressure in the anterior triangle
• What makes it a PDA?	➔ Continuous high pitched murmur in pulmonary area

3.5 Loud P$_2$

Start

Listen to the recording. This murmur was recorded in the pulmonary area in a patient with pulmonary hypertension. Focus on S$_1$ while watching the SDC and note that S$_1$ coincides with the SDC landing on systole. When confident of the timing of S$_1$, focus on S$_2$. Note that S$_2$ coincides with the SDC landing on diastole. S$_2$ is loud and crisp.

Stop

Maximize S$_2$

Start

The S$_2$ is now very loud. Make sure that you are confident of the timing of S$_2$.

Stop

Minimize S$_2$

Start

Note the phonocardiogram now without an S$_2$.

Stop

Reset

Start

Listen again to the native recording and be sure that you are confident of the timing of S$_1$ and S$_2$ and the increased intensity of S$_2$.

Chapter 4

Mid left sternal edge

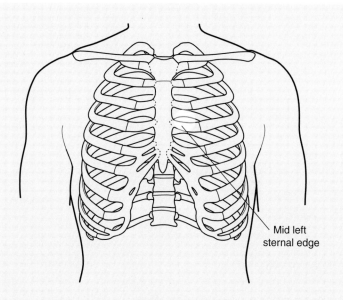

Mid left
sternal edge

The auscultatory abnormalities best heard in this region are:
- Aortic regurgitation
- Subvalvar pulmonary stenosis
- Pulmonary regurgitation
- Right bundle branch block

Aortic regurgitation

Anatomy

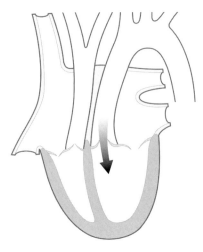

Fig. 4.1 *Aortic regurgitation*

Aortic regurgitation may occur as the predominant lesion in a congenitally bicuspid valve, or it may occur following balloon or surgical valvotomy for predominant stenosis. It may occur in a normal aortic valve as the result of aortic root dilatation or following endocarditis or rheumatic fever.

History

A bicuspid aortic valve and therefore aortic regurgitation is more common in males. Aortic regurgitation may cause shortness of breath on exertion, but if the onset is gradual the patient may be asymptomatic even in the presence of severe aortic incompetence.

Examination

There will be no abnormal cardiac physical signs in mild aortic regurgitation other than the murmur. In important aortic regurgitation there may be nailbed capillary pulsation, full volume pulses, a wide pulse pressure, a prominent left ventricular impulse and a displaced apex. In acute severe aortic regurgitation with low cardiac output the usual physical signs may be absent.

Heart sounds	S_1 normal
	S_2 Aortic component diminished
Added sounds	Nil, ejection click, S_3
Murmurs	Early diastolic decrescendo murmur

ECG

This may be normal or show voltage criteria for left ventricular hypertrophy. Repolarization changes are not uncommon in aortic regurgitation.

CXR

In mild aortic regurgitation the CXR may be normal. The cardiac silhouette may be enlarged with a left ventricular contour. There may be prominence of the ascending aorta. In acute severe aortic regurgitation there may be pulmonary oedema with minimal cardiomegaly.

Notes

There may be a soft aortic systolic ejection murmur in aortic regurgitation because of increased left ventricular stroke volume. In chronic aortic regurgitation the length and intensity of the murmur relate to the degree of aortic regurgitation. Furthermore, the more severe the regurgitation, the lower the pitch of the murmur. Important aortic regurgitation may be associated with a low pitched mid-diastolic murmur at the apex due to early partial closure of the mitral valve caused by the regurgitant jet (the Austin Flint murmur). In acute severe aortic regurgitation there may be a paucity of auscultatory findings.

Learning points
- The murmur of aortic regurgitation is decrescendo early diastolic.
- The murmur is accentuated by leaning forward and breathing out.
- Pitch as well as length and intensity relate to severity of regurgitation.
- Murmur may be absent in acute severe aortic regurgitation.

4.1 Aortic regurgitation

Start

This murmur is described as blowing and early diastolic and is maximal at the left mid sternal edge. There is no significant systolic murmur in this recording. Time the sounds with the SDC. The inexperienced auscultator often mistimes this murmur as systolic or, alternatively, does not hear it at all. We will now eliminate the diastolic component to attempt to appreciate the difference.

Stop

Minimize Diastole

Start

There is now a soft S_1 and a louder S_2. Listen to this for a few cycles and watch the SDC. Note now that there is a clear gap after S_2 where there is silence in diastole.

Stop

Maximize Diastole

Start

Focus on the SDC and note S_1 and S_2. The diastolic murmur is now loud and immediately follows S_2 and occurs when the SDC hits diastole. Compare this sound with the recording where we have again minimized diastole.

Stop

Minimize Diastole

Start

Note once more the silence after S_2. Watch the SDC to help with the timing.

Stop

Reset

Start

Finally, listen again to the native murmur and time the murmur against the SDC. You should now be able to appreciate the diastolic murmur as it was recorded.

Summary		
• Where is the murmur loudest?	→	Mid left sternal edge
• When does the murmur occur?	→	Diastole
• What else could it be?	→	Pulmonary regurgitation in the presence of pulmonary hypertension
• What makes it aortic regurgitation?	→	Pitch and position of the murmur and diastolic timing

Subvalvar pulmonary stenosis

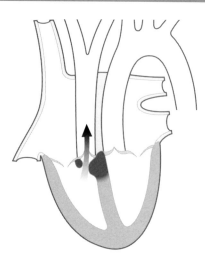

Fig. 4.2 *Subvalvar pulmonary stenosis*

Anatomy

Subvalvar pulmonary stenosis is rarely isolated, and is more commonly associated with a ventricular septal defect or as part of tetralogy of Fallot. The murmur is related to subvalvar muscle hypertrophy and/or fibrous tissue.

History

History will depend on the severity of the obstruction and the presence of associated cardiac abnormalities. The lesion is usually detected by the presence of a murmur. Severe obstruction may cause shortness of breath on exertion and chest pain.

Examination

There will be no abnormal cardiac physical signs in isolated mild subvalvar pulmonary stenosis other than the murmur. In important subvalvar stenosis there may be a palpable right ventricular impulse and thrill and even signs of right heart failure. Cyanosis may be a feature if there is a large VSD (e.g. in the tetralogy of Fallot) or an ASD.

Heart sounds	S_1 normal
	S_2 soft, normal or loud
Added sounds	Nil
Murmurs	Systolic murmur
Radiation	Pulmonary area and back

ECG

This may be normal, show right ventricular hypertrophy and possibly right ventricular strain.

CXR

In mild subvalvar pulmonary stenosis the CXR may be normal. In more severe cases there may be cardiomegaly with a right ventricular contour and reduced pulmonary vascularity. In tetralogy of Fallot there may be a right aortic arch and inconspicuous main pulmonary artery.

Notes

The second heart sound will be reduced in more severe cases. Because the stenosis is usually muscular, the obstruction and the pitch of the murmur increase during systole. In severe cases there may be complete obstruction in the latter part of systole and the murmur will become shorter and softer. In tetralogy of Fallot the aorta is anteriorly placed, so the aortic component of S_2 may be increased, and it is enlarged, so that there may also be an aortic ejection click. There will be a pulmonary ejection click if there is associated valvar pulmonary stenosis. This murmur is commonly mistaken for a VSD but the murmur of subpulmonary stenosis often radiates to the pulmonary area and through to the back.

Learning point
- The murmur of subpulmonary stenosis may be similar to a VSD.

4.2 Pulmonary stenosis (subvalvar)

Start

Listen to the recording. This is a 2/6 ejection systolic murmur recorded at the mid left sternal edge. Watch the SDC and note that the murmur coincides with it hitting systole. Try to appreciate S_1 and S_2. S_1 is very quiet and S_2 is clear. This murmur could be described as soft, early systolic and occupying three-quarters of systole (hence S_1 is masked by the murmur and S_2 is not). There is no click. We shall now manipulate the heart sounds.

Stop

Maximize Systole

Start

You have increased the intensity of the systolic murmur. Watch the SDC and time the heart sounds and the murmur.

Stop

Minimize Systole

Start

Listen and note that the systolic murmur has almost disappeared. S_2 is clear and is widely split.

Stop

Reset

Start

Listen to the native murmur. Note the very soft S_1, the clearly audible and split S_2 and the soft systolic murmur.

Summary		
• Where is the murmur loudest?	→	Mid left sternal edge
• When does the murmur occur?	→	Systole
• What else could it be?	→	Ventricular septal defect
• What makes it subvalvar pulmonary stenosis?	→	Radiation to the back and rising pitch in systole

Pulmonary regurgitation

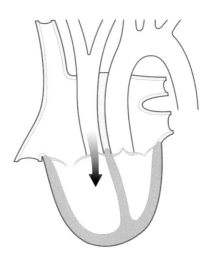

Fig. 4.3 *Pulmonary regurgitation*

Anatomy

Isolated pulmonary regurgitation is rare. More commonly pulmonary regurgitation is present after surgery for pulmonary stenosis, particularly in the setting of tetralogy of Fallot.

History

As noted above, there may be a history of surgical or cardiac catheter treatment of a stenotic pulmonary valve. In isolated congenital pulmonary regurgitation, the patient is often symptomatic well into adult life. Pulmonary hypertension may cause pulmonary regurgitation.

Examination

In mild pulmonary regurgitation the examination will be normal apart from the presence of a murmur. In important pulmonary regurgitation there will be a right ventricular impulse. Right ventricular failure is rare but may occur with chronic severe regurgitation and lead to elevation in the central venous pressure, hepatomegaly and oedema.

Heart sounds	S$_1$ normal
	S$_2$ often widely split
Added sounds	Nil, or pulmonary ejection click
Murmurs	Medium- to low-pitched diastolic crescendo–decrescendo murmur

ECG

The ECG is usually normal. There may be signs of right ventricular volume overload. Following surgery for tetralogy of Fallot there will usually be complete right bundle branch block.

CXR

This may be normal. Often there is dilatation of the pulmonary trunk. With severe regurgitation there will be enlargement of the right ventricle.

Notes

The second heart sound is usually widely split due to delay in the pulmonary component, often with right bundle branch block; however, the second heart sound may be single in complete absence of the pulmonary valve. The second heart sound may be closely split if rapid right ventricular ejection is accompanied by a rapid fall in pulmonary artery pressure.

The murmur is typically mid-diastolic and short in duration. However, in pulmonary hypertension there is a large pressure difference throughout diastole and the murmur is high pitched, and long, sometimes lasting throughout diastole (Graham Steell murmur).

Learning points
- Pulmonary hypertension may cause pulmonary regurgitation in the presence of a normal pulmonary valve.
- Pulmonary regurgitation is common after repair of tetralogy of Fallot.

))) **4.3 Pulmonary regurgitation**

Start

There is a soft systolic and diastolic murmur recorded at the left mid sternal edge. This is the area that pulmonary regurgitation is best heard. It is vital to be able to hear the two components of the murmur separately. Most trainees initially perceive the systolic murmur but cannot hear the diastolic component. We will now eliminate the diastolic component to hear the difference.

Stop

Minimize Diastole

Start

There is now a soft S_1, a soft ejection systolic murmur and a louder S_2. Listen to this for a few cycles and note that there is a clear gap after S_2 where there is silence (i.e. diastole).

Stop

Maximize Diastole

Start

Focus on the two heart sounds and try to appreciate the murmur after S_2 (when the cursor hits diastole). This is the diastolic component, which is short and early. Start this and then compare it with the murmur when you have again minimized diastole.

Stop

Minimize Diastole

Start

Note again the silence after S_2, which is now once again the end of the murmur. If you are still having difficulty in appreciating the diastolic murmur on the native recording try the following.

Stop

Maximize Diastole and Minimize Systole

Start

The systolic murmur has almost disappeared and the diastolic murmur is accentuated. Watch the SDC and time the murmur: it is clear that the louder murmur is diastolic.

Stop

Reset

Start

Listen finally to the native murmur and time again with the SDC. You should now be able to appreciate both parts of the murmur.

4.4 Pulmonary regurgitation with pulmonary hypertension

Start

Listen to the recording. There is a diastolic murmur recorded at the left mid sternal edge, where the murmur of pulmonary regurgitation is best heard. In the presence of pulmonary hypertension the diastolic murmur of pulmonary regurgitation is higher pitched and can be impossible to differentiate from the murmur of aortic regurgitation. As with all diastolic murmurs, the timing is not immediately apparent and we will now manipulate the diastolic component to help appreciate it.

Stop

Minimize Diastole

Start

Watch the SDC. Note that there is now silence in diastole, with S_2 marking the beginning of the silence.

Stop

Maximize Diastole

Start

The diastolic murmur is now really quite loud and dominates the sounds. Listen carefully while watching the SDC. To ensure that the timing of the murmur is appreciated, we shall now eliminate it again.

Stop

Minimise Diastole

Start

Note again the silence after S_2. Watch the SDC while listening.

Stop

Reset

Start

Listen to the native murmur. Watch the SDC and time the murmur.

Summary	
• Where is the murmur loudest?	➔ Mid left sternal edge
• When does the murmur occur?	➔ Diastole
• What else could it be?	➔ Aortic regurgitation, in the absence of pulmonary hypertension, pulmonary regurgitation is usually lower pitched
• What makes it pulmonary regurgitation?	➔ Diastolic timing and quality

⚙ 4.5 Right bundle branch block

Start

Listen carefully. There is a very soft systolic murmur and there is wide splitting of S_2. Splitting of the second sound, even when it is wide, is a subtle finding. Note that the split S_2 occurs as the SDC hits diastole.

Stop

Minimize Systole

Start

You have eliminated the very soft systolic murmur and can now focus your attention on S_2. Try to appreciate the splitting and don't worry, it is not that obvious.

Stop

Maximize S_2 Split

Start

Listen carefully and focus on S_2. The systolic murmur is quiet and we have widened the splitting, making it easier to appreciate.

Stop

Minimize S_2 Split

Start

Listen carefully; watch the SDC. The second sound remains somewhat split, but less so than previously.

Stop

Reset

Start

Listen to the native recording and be sure that you appreciate the splitting of S_2.

Chapter 5

Lower left sternal edge

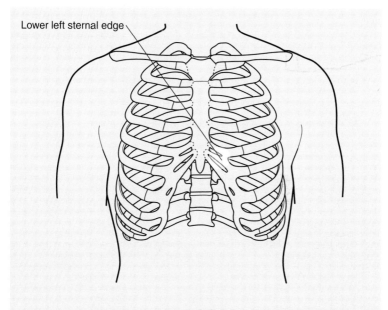

Lower left sternal edge

The murmurs best heard in this region are:
- Innocent vibratory murmur
- Ventricular septal defect
- Subaortic stenosis
- Tricuspid regurgitation

Innocent vibratory (Still's) murmur

Anatomy

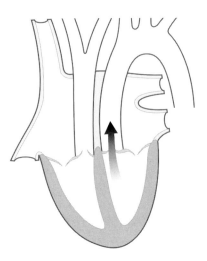

Fig. 5.1 *Innocent vibratory murmur*

This is a very common innocent murmur, most often heard from 3 years of age to adolescence, and by definition the anatomy is normal. The origin of this murmur is uncertain but it may arise from the left ventricular outflow tract.

History

Since the heart is normal, there can be no symptoms attributable to the heart.

Examination

General and cardiac examination is normal apart from the murmur.

Heart sounds	Normal
Added sounds	Normal
Murmurs	Early systolic vibratory murmur

ECG
The ECG is normal.

CXR
The CXR will be normal.

Notes

Innocent vibratory murmurs have a very distinctive sound that has been compared to the twanging of a rubber band. They may be quite loud, up to grade 3/6, but are never associated with a thrill.

Learning points
- Innocent murmurs are very common in childhood.
- Classical vibratory murmurs are very distinctive. Occasionally, however, a soft vibratory murmur may be very difficult to differentiate from mild subaortic stenosis.

5.1 Vibratory systolic murmur

Start

Listen to the recording. The vibratory murmur is one of the 'innocent' murmurs of childhood, otherwise known as the Still's murmur. It is loudest at the lower left or mid left sternal edge. Watch the SDC and note that the murmur coincides with it hitting systole and is very soft (1/6 in intensity). Try to appreciate S_1 and S_2, which are clearly and discretely audible. The main diagnostic feature of this murmur is its quality. We shall now manipulate the heart sounds.

Stop

Maximize Systole

Start

You have maximized this murmur: if you could not hear it before, it should be more apparent now. S_1 is also now softer than S_2. Watch the SDC and time the two heart sounds.

Stop

Minimize Systole

Start

Listen and note the absence of the systolic murmur. In case you still have problems we will now maximize and minimize the murmur again to help you to appeciate it.

Stop

Maximize Systole

Start

Listen and appreciate the 'absence of nothing' in systole.

Stop

Minimize Systole

Start

Listen again to the silence in systole.

Stop

Reset

Start

Listen to the native murmur and be sure you can appreciate a soft vibratory murmur.

Summary		
• Where is the murmur loudest?	→	Lower left sternal edge
• When does the murmur occur?	→	Systole
• What else could it be?	→	Ventricular septal defect or subaortic stenosis
• What makes it a Still's murmur?	→	Position of the murmur, absence of thrill, and quality of the murmur

Ventricular septal defect

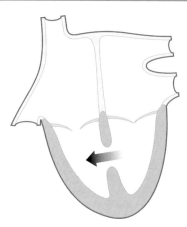

Fig. 5.2 *Ventricular septal defect*

Anatomy

A ventricular septal defect (VSD) is a hole in the septum between the two ventricles. VSDs may vary in size from pinhole to almost complete absence of the septum, and the physical signs vary accordingly. The position of the defect is usually perimembranous (around the membranous septum adjacent to the aortic and tricuspid valves) or muscular (anywhere else).

History

The presentation of a VSD will depend upon its size. Small defects are diagnosed because of a murmur heard on routine examination. Larger defects cause 'heart failure'.

Examination

There may be no abnormal cardiac physical signs in a small VSD other than a cardiac murmur, although a thrill is not uncommon. In moderate defects there will be signs of left ventricular volume overload, including a prominent left ventricular impulse which may be displaced, and a mitral diastolic flow murmur. Large defects may present with heart failure in infancy and may cause pulmonary hypertension, the signs of which may then predominate.

Small ventricular septal defect

Heart sounds	S_1 normal
	S_2 normal
Added sounds	Nil
Murmurs	Pansystolic murmur, or early systolic murmur if smaller

Moderate ventricular septal defect

Heart sounds	S_1 normal
	S_2 normal or accentuated
Added sounds	Nil, third heart sound
Murmurs	Systole: pansystolic murmur
	Diastole: mitral flow murmur

ECG

The ECG will be normal in small defects, but will demonstrate voltage criteria for left ventricular or biventricular hypertrophy in medium to large defects. With the onset of pulmonary hypertension, right ventricular hypertrophy will predominate.

CXR

This will be normal in small defects. Moderate defects will cause left atrial and left ventricular dilatation with pulmonary plethora. Radiological evidence of pulmonary hypertension may supervene.

Notes

As a VSD becomes smaller the murmur becomes shorter because the defect closes before the end of systole. In moderate VSDs with large left to right shunts there may be mid-systolic accentuation of the murmur due to a pulmonary flow component, and similarly there may be a mitral diastolic flow murmur. Perimembranous VSDs may be associated with aortic regurgitation. Subaortic stenosis may cause a similar murmur to a small VSD but radiates to the aortic area. Similarly, subpulmonary stenosis may be confused with a VSD but the murmur radiates to the pulmonary area and through to the back. The murmur of tricuspid regurgitation is similar to that of a small VSD.

Learning points
- Subaortic stenosis may masquerade as a VSD.
- Perimembranous VSDs may be associated with aortic regurgitation.
- Small VSDs may cause a loud murmur.
- Large VSDs may only cause a soft murmur.

5.2 Loud muscular ventricular septal defect

Start

Listen to this murmur. It is described as a blowing systolic murmur of 3–4/6 intensity which occupies three-quarters of systole. Watch the SDC and note that the murmur coincides with it hitting systole. Try to appreciate S_2, which is clearly audible (i.e. the murmur does not run into S_2 and therefore the murmur is not pansystolic). We shall now manipulate the heart sounds.

Stop

Minimize Systole

Start

You have *greatly diminished* the systolic murmur and you can focus on the heart sounds. S_1 is slightly softer than S_2. Watch the SDC and time the two heart sounds.

Stop

Maximize S_2

Start

Listen and note the louder S_2.

Stop

Minimize S_2 and maximize Systole

Start

Note the systolic murmur and that S_2 is now inaudible. Because S_2 is now inaudible the murmur sounds pansystolic. (Murmurs in VSDs are often described in textbooks as pansystolic, but this is not always the case.)

Stop

Reset

Start

Listen to the native murmur and again confirm that the murmur does not in fact reach S_2, which is clearly audible. Remember—not all VSD murmurs are pansystolic!

5.3 Very small muscular ventricular septal defect

Start

Listen to the recording. This is a blowing systolic murmur of 2/6 intensity which occupies three-quarters of systole. Watch the SDC and note that the murmur coincides with it hitting systole. Try to appreciate S_2, which is clearly audible (i.e. the murmur does not run into S_2 and therefore the murmur is not pansystolic). We shall now manipulate the heart sounds.

Stop

Minimize Systole

Start

You have eliminated the systolic murmur and you can focus on the heart sounds. S_1 is slightly softer than S_2. Watch the SDC and time the two heart sounds.

Stop

Maximize S_2

Start

Listen and note louder S_2.

Stop

Minimise S_2 and maximize Systole

Start

Note the louder systolic murmur and that S_2 is inaudible. Because S_2 is now inaudible the murmur sounds pansystolic (as in the classical description of a VSD murmur).

Stop

Reset

Start

Listen to the native murmur and again confirm that the murmur does not in fact reach S_2, which is clearly audible. *Use this case to learn to separate the murmur from S_2 when possible—not all VSD murmurs are pansystolic!*

5.4 Perimembranous ventricular septal defect

Start

Listen to the recording. This is a blowing systolic murmur of 3–4/6 intensity which occupies three-quarters of systole. Watch the SDC and note that the murmur coincides with it hitting systole. Try to appreciate S_2, which is clearly audible. (The murmur does not run into S_2 and therefore the murmur is not pansystolic. The classical teaching is that the murmur of a perimembranous VSD is pansystolic but this is by no means always the case). We shall now manipulate the heart sounds.

Stop

Minimize Systole

Start

You have eliminated the systolic murmur and you can focus on the heart sounds. S_1 is slightly softer than S_2. Watch the SDC and time the two heart sounds.

Stop

Maximize S_2

Start

Listen and note louder S_2.

Stop

Minimize S_2 and maximize Systole

Start

Note the systolic murmur and that S_2 is inaudible. Because S_2 is now inaudible the murmur sounds pansystolic.

Stop

Reset

Start

Listen to the native murmur and again confirm that the murmur does not in fact reach S_2, which is clearly audible. Use this case to learn to separate the murmur from S_2 when possible—not all VSD murmurs are pansystolic!

Summary	
• Where is the murmur loudest?	→ Lower left sternal edge
• When does the murmur occur?	→ Systole
• What else could it be?	→ Subvalvar pulmonary or aortic stenosis, innocent Still's murmur
• What makes it a VSD?	→ Quality of the murmur

Subaortic stenosis

Anatomy

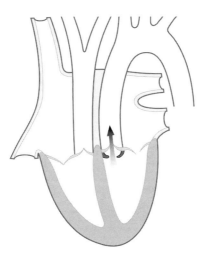

Fig. 5.3 *Subaortic stenosis*

Subaortic stenosis is most commonly caused by a fibrous cresent-shaped membrane, although a longer fibromuscular tunnel is not uncommon. It may be isolated, or associated with other congenital abnormalities, particularly an abnormal aortic or mitral valve, and in association with a VSD.

History

Subaortic stenosis is rare in infancy, and commonest in childhood and young adulthood. The patient may be asymptomatic despite severe obstruction, although tiredness on exercise and syncope on exercise are worrying symptoms. Angina is not uncommon in important obstruction.

Examination

In mild obstruction the examination will be normal apart from the presence of a murmur. The arterial pulse may be of small volume in important subaortic obstruction. There may also be a thrill in the suprasternal notch and over the carotid arteries, and this may be present at the mid left sternal edge (mimicking that of a VSD). In severe obstruction there may be a left ventricular heave.

Heart sounds	S$_1$ normal
	S$_2$ normal or soft
Added sounds	Nil
Murmurs	Long systolic murmur which radiates to the aortic area

ECG

The ECG is normal in mild obstruction. Left ventricular forces are increased in important obstruction and there may be repolarization changes.

CXR

This may be normal even with severe obstruction.

Notes

The aortic component of the second sound becomes quieter as the degree of obstruction increases.

Learning points
- Aortic regurgitation is present in about 50% of cases.
- Subaortic obstruction may be progressive.
- Subaortic obstruction may be confused with a VSD.

🔵 5.5 Aortic stenosis – subvalvar

Start

Note the systolic murmur, which in subaortic stenosis is loudest at the lower left sternal edge (the murmur of valvar aortic stenosis is loudest in the aortic area). It is blowing and long but does not reach S_2, which is clearly heard.

Stop

Minimize S_2

Start

Note that the second sound has now gone and the murmur is not unlike the pansystolic murmur of certain types of VSD. In fact this murmur is now indistinguishable from a VSD murmur.

Stop

Maximize S_2

Start

Confirm that S_2 is clearly audible after the end of the murmur.

Stop

Minimize Systole

Start

The murmur is now very quiet and the heart sounds are clearly audible.

Stop

Reset

Start

Listen to the native murmur and note the features described.

Summary

• Where is the murmur loudest?	→ Lower left sternal edge
• When does the murmur occur?	→ Systole
• What else could it be?	→ Innocent murmur, VSD, tricuspid regurgitation
• What makes it subaortic stenosis?	→ Radiation to aortic area

Tricuspid regurgitation

Anatomy

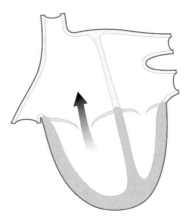

Fig. 5.4 *Tricuspid regurgitation*

Isolated tricuspid regurgitation is most common with Ebstein's anomaly of the tricuspid valve, in which the septal leaflet of the valve is attached further down the ventricular septum than normal. The degree of tricuspid regurgitation ranges from mild to torrential. Tricuspid regurgitation may result from a dysplastic valve and occasionally after spontaneous closure of a VSD when the septal leaflet becomes adherent to the margins of the defect. Tricuspid regurgitation may also occur if an anatomically normal valve becomes stretched as a result of right heart dilatation, for example, due to an atrial septal defect or after surgery for tetralogy of Fallot.

History

Severe tricuspid regurgitation may lead to fetal hydrops or even death in utero. The patient may present in early infancy with cyanosis, breathlessness and low cardiac output. In less severe cases the diagnosis may be made because of the murmur, the presence of cyanosis, which may deepen with time, or palpitations or syncope due to atrial arrhythmias. Patients may, however, be asymptomatic well into adult life.

Examination

There may be central cyanosis. Some patients have ruddy cheeks. The jugular venous pulse is (surprisingly) normal until right ventricular failure occurs. In Ebstein's anomaly there may be no right ventricular heave, but this is usually present when tricuspid regurgitation is due to other causes.

Heart sounds	S_1 normal or loud and single in Ebstein's anomaly
	S_2 normal or may be widely split
Added sounds	Nil, S_3 and S_4 may be heard
Murmurs	Early systolic/pansystolic murmur

ECG

The PR interval may be short, normal or prolonged. Pre-excitation is present in 25% of patients with Ebstein's anomaly and the P wave is usually tall. The QRS complex is usually prolonged and shows a right bundle branch block pattern.

CXR

The cardiac contour may be normal or enlarged, sometimes massively so. The pulmonary vascularity is either normal or decreased. The pulmonary trunk is inconspicuous in Ebstein's anomaly, but will be enlarged if the tricuspid regurgitation is the result of an ASD or is associated with pulmonary regurgitation.

Notes

The murmur can vary in length from early systolic to pansystolic.

Summary	
• Where is the murmur loudest?	➔ Lower left sternal edge
• When does the murmur occur?	➔ Systole
• What else could it be?	➔ VSD or subaortic stenosis
• What makes it tricuspid regurgitation?	➔ Quality and variation with respiration

Chapter 6

Apex

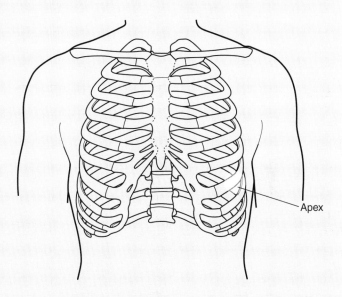

The apex is between the mid-clavicular line and the anterior axillary line in the fifth intercostal space on the left.

The murmurs best heard in this region are:
- Mitral regurgitation
- Mitral valve prolapse
- Mitral valve stenosis

Mitral regurgitation

Anatomy

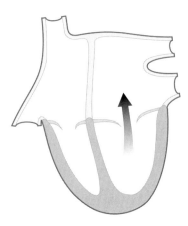

Fig. 6.1   *Mitral regurgitation*

Isolated mitral regurgitation is rare in childhood, and in paediatric practice it is usually associated with atrioventricular septal defects. In adulthood it is more common and often associated with ischaemic heart disease in the setting of reduced left ventricular function, when it is often referred to as 'functional' mitral regurgitation resulting from mitral annular dilatation. Other causes include rheumatic valve disease, mitral valve dysplasia, congenital clefts in the mitral valve leaflets (usually the anterior leaflet) and in association with parachute mitral valve. When mitral regurgitation is present, the left ventricle becomes volume loaded (i.e. there is an increase in pre-load) because the ventricle has to accommodate, in diastole, the normal pulmonary venous return plus the regurgitant volume. The left ventricular end diastolic volume increases and, if unchecked, can lead to myocardial dysfunction. The aim of follow-up is to intervene before this stage is reached.

History

Mild to moderate mitral regurgitation is not usually associated with symptoms but effort intolerance and breathlessness will supervene as it progresses.

Examination

On examination, in mild cases, the murmur will be the only abnormal cardiac physical sign. As the degree of mitral regurgitation progresses a prominent apical impulse will be apparent and this will become displaced towards and beyond the anterior axillary line in more severe cases. Severe mitral regurgitation is a cause of congestive cardiac failure, which will be manifest by the usual signs and symptoms.

Heart sounds	Normal
Added sounds	None, S_3, S_4, $S_3 + S_4$ (gallop rhythm)
Murmurs	Systolic (not 'ejection')
	Associated diastolic murmur in severe cases

ECG

The ECG is usually normal in mild to moderate mitral regurgitation but, as the severity increases, voltage criteria for left ventricular hypertrophy may develop. Repolarization abnormalities (ST depression and T wave inversion in the inferolateral leads) may be associated with important mitral regurgitation.

CXR

This will be normal in mild mitral regurgitation. As the degree of mitral regurgitation becomes haemodynamically significant, the left atrium will enlarge and be associated with splaying of the carina. The left ventricular contour will become more prominent (a 'rounding off' of the apex) and cardiomegaly will be apparent.

Notes

The murmur of mitral regurgitation is systolic and starts at the onset of systole (compare this to the special case of mitral regurgitation associated with mitral valve prolapse, when the murmur may be late systolic). The intensity relates reasonably well to the severity, but be aware that severe mitral regurgitation can be associated with a quiet murmur, particularly when there is left ventricular dysfunction. The murmur can occupy any proportion of systole but is classically described as a 'pansystolic' or 'holosystolic' murmur. The less severe the mitral regurgitation the shorter the murmur tends to be, so that in very mild cases it will be soft and early systolic. If left ventricular dysfunction supervenes, added sounds will appear and eventually a gallop rhythm may develop. In moderate and severe cases of mitral regurgitation there is increased *diastolic* flow across the mitral valve and, as a result, an apical mitral *diastolic* murmur may be heard which is similar to that associated with mitral stenosis.

Learning points
- The murmur of mitral regurgitation begins with S_1.
- The murmur of mitral regurgitation is classically but not necessarily pansystolic.
- A soft murmur does not always represent mild disease.
- A mitral diastolic murmur (in the absence of mitral stenosis) indicates important regurgitation.
- Acute severe mitral regurgitation causes pulmonary oedema and a murmur may be absent.

6.1 Mitral regurgitation

Start

Listen to the recording. There is a soft systolic murmur representing mild mitral regurgitation. S_1 is audible and coincides with the SDC hitting 'Systole'. The murmur begins just after S_1. S_2 marks the end of the murmur. Try to appreciate the murmur before we reduce its intensity.

Stop

Minimize Systole

Start

The heart sounds are clear but the murmur has disappeared. As you listen, watch the SDC to time the heart sounds.

Stop

Maximize Systole

Start

The murmur is now louder and is still typical of mitral regurgitation.

Stop

Reset

Start

Listen to the native murmur and continue to time it by watching the SDC.

Summary		
• Where is the murmur loudest?	→	Apex
• When does the murmur occur?	→	Systole
• What else could it be?	→	VSD
• What makes it mitral regurgitation?	→	Position at the apex

Mitral valve prolapse

Anatomy

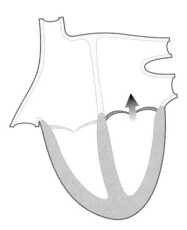

Fig. 6.2 *Mitral valve prolapse*

Mitral valve prolapse is a specific disorder of the mitral valve papillary muscles resulting in a lack of support of one or both leaflets and varying degrees of mitral regurgitation. It is more common in females and the overall incidence is probably around 1% but depends on the criteria used to define prolapse. It is also more common in connective tissue disorders, such as Ehlers–Danlos syndrome, and may be seen in Marfan syndrome, when it may be associated with aortic root dilatation.

History

It has been suggested that atypical chest pain is more common in people with mitral valve prolapse. Rare patients with mitral valve prolapse will develop acute rupture. Symptoms will depend on the degree and rate of progression of regurgitation and the notes above will equally apply here.

Examination

There is frequently a systolic click reflecting the prolapse, and the murmur of mitral regurgitation immediately follows this. The classical case will therefore have an apical systolic click and late systolic murmur. However, in minor cases there will be a click without a murmur, making it difficult to differentiate it from the ejection click associated with a bicuspid aortic valve, which is also often loudest at the apex. Furthermore, severe mitral valve prolapse may be associated with a pansystolic murmur of mitral regurgitation without a click: echocardiography is necessary to make the diagnosis of mitral valve prolapse in these cases. See notes above on mitral regurgitation.

Heart sounds	Normal
Added sounds	None, systolic click, S_3, S_4, $S_3 + S_4$ (gallop rhythm)
Murmurs	None, late systolic or pansystolic
	Associated diastolic murmur in severe cases

ECG
As for mitral regurgitation.

CXR
As for mitral regurgitation.

Learning points
- Mitral valve prolapse is a specific cause of mitral regurgitation.
- Mitral valve prolapse is usually associated with an apical systolic click and late systolic murmur.
- Mitral valve prolapse can present with acute rupture.
- Look for signs of the Marfan syndrome and other connective tissue disorders.

6.2 Mitral valve prolapse with ejection click and soft systolic murmur

Start

Listen to the recording. This is an example of mitral valve prolapse, but in this case there is a click. The click follows S_1 and can be mistaken for a split S_1. There is a soft systolic murmur which begins towards the end of systole, the typical late systolic murmur of mitral valve prolapse. S_2 marks the end of the murmur. To appreciate the systolic click and murmur we will now reduce the intensity of systole.

Stop

Minimize Systole

Start

The heart sounds are clear but the click and murmur have disappeared. As you listen, watch the SDC to time the heart sounds.

Stop

Maximize Systole

Start

The systolic click and murmur are now reasonably loud.

Stop

Reset

Start

Listen to the native click and murmur and continue to time them by watching the SDC.

Summary	
• Where is the murmur loudest?	→ Apex
• When does the murmur occur?	→ Systole
• What else could it be?	→ The click could be from the aortic valve; the murmur could be a ventricular septal defect
• What makes it mitral valve prolapse?	→ The association of a click and murmur, loudest at the apex

Mitral valve stenosis

Anatomy

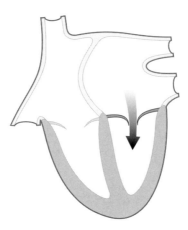

Fig. 6.3 *Mitral valve stenosis*

Mitral valve stenosis is usually rheumatic in origin and associated with mitral regurgitation. It is becoming less common in adult practice in the West. In childhood it is extremely rare and results from congenital abnormalities of the mitral valve (e.g. parachute mitral valve). It is also sometimes seen following repair of atrioventricular septal defects when there is residual mitral valve dysfunction.

History

As with all valvar lesions, if the degree of mitral stenosis is mild there will be no symptoms and the only signs will be on auscultation. As the degree of stenosis and/or regurgitation progresses, effort dyspnoea will develop. The rate of progression of the disease will vary but in severe cases symptoms of congestive cardiac failure will develop.

Examination

The so-called 'mitral facies' is a feature of chronic severe mitral stenosis. Effort dyspnoea may occur and haemoptysis may be a presenting feature. Because of the elevated left atrial pressure there is often a degree of pulmonary hypertension, reflected by a prominent right ventricular impulse and a loud second sound. In severe cases of mitral stenosis there may be an apical *diastolic* thrill that is easy to mistime as systolic without careful comparison with a central pulse.

Heart sounds	Loud S_1
	Loud S_2 (if pulmonary hypertension)
Added sounds	Opening snap, S_4
Murmurs	Mitral stenosis: apical mid-diastolic, rumbling with presystolic accentuation (if sinus rhythm)
	Mitral regurgitation: apical long or pansystolic murmur
	Murmur of pulmonary regurgitation if severe pulmonary hypertension supervenes

ECG

The ECG is usually abnormal in significant mitral stenosis. There is generally evidence of left atrial hypertrophy, and if pulmonary hypertension supervenes there will be voltage criteria for right ventricular hypertrophy.

CXR

This may be normal in very mild disease. Significant disease will cause prominence of the left atrium with splaying of the carina. Pulmonary venous hypertension will be reflected by prominent upper lobe veins. The enlarged left atrium causes prominence of the appendage and straightening of the left heart border. There may be calcification in the region of the mitral valve, notably in rheumatic mitral stenosis. In severe disease, as pulmonary arterial hypertension develops, there will be prominence of the central pulmonary arteries with, in advanced cases, peripheral arterial pruning.

Notes

The murmurs of mitral valve disease are loudest at the apex and are accentuated by lying the patient on the left side and listening with the bell of the stethoscope.

In a case of mixed mitral disease it is important to be able to make an assessment of the haemodynamic importance of each: if the dominant lesion is stenosis, the heart will not be enlarged on palpation, there may be a diastolic thrill, the P_2 may be palpable, and the murmur will be loudest in diastole. Don't forget the late diastolic (pre-systolic) accentuation caused by the active phase of left ventricular filling secondary to atrial systole.

If the dominant lesion is regurgitation, the apex will be displaced and thrusting and the dominant murmur will be systolic. Remember that if regurgitation is important the diastolic murmur may be accentuated because of the resulting increased diastolic flow across the mitral valve: a mitral diastolic murmur can even develop when there is no stenosis (see mitral regurgitation above).

Learning points

- It is possible to assess which lesion is dominant in mixed mitral valve disease.
- A *diastolic* thrill in mitral stenosis is easy to mistime as *systolic*.

6.3 Mitral stenosis and regurgitation

Start

Listen to the recording. There is a soft systolic murmur and a soft diastolic murmur. The systolic murmur is the murmur of mild mitral regurgitation. The diastolic murmur is that of mild mitral stenosis. The murmurs of mitral stenosis and regurgitation are both loudest at the apex, where this recording was made. Time the sounds with the SDC. The mitral regurgitation obviously coincides with the SDC hitting systole, and the mitral stenosis with the cursor hitting diastole. We will now eliminate the diastolic component to attempt to hear the difference.

Stop

Minimize Diastole

Start

S_1 is very soft and S_2 is prominent. Listen to the systolic murmur for a few cycles and note that there is nothing after S_2 (during diastole). Watch the SDC while listening. Get the timing of each part of the cardiac cycle. Become familiar with the period of 'nothing' during diastole. It is the absence of 'nothing' that you will hear next.

Stop

Maximize Diastole

Start

Focus on S_1 (almost inaudible) and S_2 and watch the SDC. Note the systolic murmur. Note now the 'absence of nothing' when the SDC hits diastole. This is the diastolic murmur of mitral stenosis. It is described as low pitched and rumbling. Listen carefully for as long as it takes to appreciate fully this part of the murmur. You may also be able to appreciate the presystolic accentuation caused by atrial systole just before S_1. If you are still having difficulty differentiating the systolic murmur from the diastolic murmur, move on to the next stage.

Stop

Minimize Systole

Start

Note that there is now no systolic murmur. Watch the SDC and note that the murmur is purely diastolic, with all the features described above.

Stop

Maximize Systole

Start

Both the systolic and diastolic murmurs are set at maximum intensity. Listen until you are confident that you are clearly separating the two components.

Stop

Reset

Start

Listen finally to the native murmurs, and time again with the SDC. You should now be able to appreciate both parts of the murmur in its unaltered form.

Summary	
• Where is the murmur loudest?	→ Apex
• When does the murmur occur?	→ Diastole (stenosis) and systole (regurgitation)
• What else could it be?	→ Nothing
• What makes it mitral stenosis and mitral regurgitation?	→ Timing and position of the murmur

6.4 Mitral stenosis (opening snap)

Start

This is a recording of pure mild mitral stenosis and was recorded at the apex, S_1 is loud but the diastolic murmur of mitral stenosis in this case is soft. The opening snap is a prominent feature. Time the sounds with the SDC. The opening snap follows very soon after S_2 and can indeed be confused with splitting of S_2. We will now minimize the diastolic sounds, which will eliminate both the opening snap and the soft diastolic murmur.

Stop

Minimize Diastole

Start

S_1 remains prominent and S_2 is soft. Listen to the sound for a few cycles and note that there is nothing after S_2 (during diastole). Watch the SDC while listening. Get the timing of each part of the cardiac cycle. Become familiar with the period of 'nothing' during diastole. It is the 'absence of nothing' that you will hear next.

Stop

Maximize Diastole

Start

Focus on S_1 and S_2 and watch the SDC. Note the opening snap after S_2 and the diastolic murmur which immediately follows it. Note now the 'absence of nothing' when the SDC hits diastole. To be sure that the opening snap and diastolic murmur are being appreciated, we will now reduce its intensity again.

Stop

Minimize Diastole

Start

S_1 remains prominent and S_2 is soft. Listen to the sound for a few cycles and note that there is nothing after S_2 (during diastole). Watch the SDC while listening. Get the timing of each part of the cardiac cycle. Become familiar with the period of 'nothing' during diastole. It is the 'absence of nothing' that you will hear next.

Stop

Reset

Start

Listen finally to the native murmur and time again with the SDC. You should now be able to appreciate clearly the opening snap, although the diastolic murmur is soft.

Chapter 7

The Back

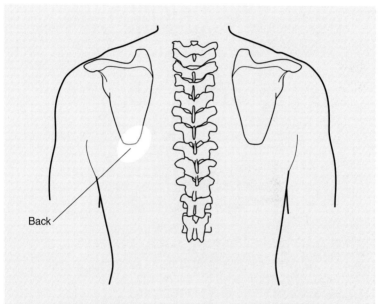

Back

A few murmurs are not just transmitted to the back of the chest but are actually louder there.

The murmurs best heard at the back are:
- Coarctation
- Branch pulmonary artery stenosis

Coarctation

Anatomy

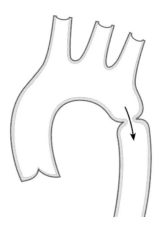

Fig. 7.1   *Coarctation*

Coarctation of the aorta may be isolated or may be associated with abnormalities of the aortic valve, mitral valve and the aortic arch. We will only consider isolated coarctation.

History

Patients will often be asymptomatic. The most common symptoms will be as a result of associated hypertension.

Examination

Palpation of the femoral pulses will show low volume or completely absent pulses. The left brachial pulse may be normal or low volume depending on the relationship of the coarctation to the left subclavian artery. There may be visible pulsation in the neck. The blood pressure will often be elevated in the right arm.

Heart sounds	Normal
Added sounds	Nil, unless associated with valvar heart disease
Murmurs	Ejection systolic murmur over left side of chest; continuous murmur over posterior chest wall (collaterals)

ECG

This will often be normal but may show left ventricular hypertrophy because of hypertension.

CXR

There may be cardiomegaly. The aortic arch shadow may be inconspicuous. There may be a '3 sign'. At the left upper border there is prominence of the arch just proximal to the narrow segment and post-stenotic dilatation just beyond. In adults and older children with good collateral arterial supply there may be rib notching.

Notes

There will often be an aortic ejection click at the apex, possibly with an aortic systolic murmur due to the frequent association of a bicuspid aortic valve.

Learning points
- Always measure blood pressure, feel the femoral pulses and compare with radial pulses.
- Weak femoral pulses do not necessarily indicate peripheral vascular disease.

Summary		
• Where is the murmur loudest?	➜	At the back
• When does the murmur occur?	➜	Systole
• What else could it be?	➜	Branch pulmonary artery stenosis
• What makes it coarctation?	➜	Presence of poor femoral pulses

Branch pulmonary artery stenosis

Anatomy

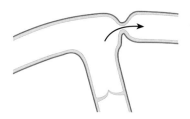

Fig. 7.2 *Branch pulmonary artery stenosis*

In the newborn infant, particularly premature babies and those who are small at birth, it is very common to hear a murmur arising from the origin of either pulmonary artery. This disappears as the pulmonary arteries grow over the first few months of life.

True narrowings at the origins of either pulmonary artery, or further out in the pulmonary arterial tree, are relatively frequent in association with tetralogy of Fallot. Pulmonary arterial abnormalities may occur in association with Williams syndrome, Alagille syndrome and fetal rubella.

History

Patients will often be asymptomatic, although breathlessness on exertion may be a feature.

Examination

If stenoses are bilateral and severe, there may be signs of right ventricular hypertrophy, with a right ventricular heave, and eventually right ventricular failure, with a raised jugular venous pressure, hepatomegaly and peripheral oedema.

Heart sounds	Normal
Added sounds	Nil
Murmurs	Ejection systolic murmurs over the affected lung(s)

ECG

There may be signs of right ventricular hypertrophy, although these may be absent, even in the presence of a significantly raised right ventricular pressure.

CXR

If the stenosis is unilateral, there may be a difference in the pulmonary vascular markings visible on comparing the two lungs. In multiple peripheral stenoses, the overall pulmonary vascularity may be decreased. The cardiac contour is often normal until the onset of right ventricular failure.

Notes

Branch pulmonary artery murmurs are often audible over the whole precordium, but are louder posteriorly over the lung fields. Rarely, there may be a diastolic component due to diastolic forward flow in severe cases.

Glossary

Arrhythmia: Abnormally fast or slow heart heart rate.

Ascites: Free fluid in the abdominal cavity. May occur in severe cardiac failure.

Bell chestpiece: Part of stethoscope designed to detect low frequency sounds.

Cyanosis: Blueness. This may be peripheral, affecting the extremities, which is normal in the cold and is common in children, or central, affecting the lips and tongue as well as the extremities, and indicates a low arterial oxygen tension.

Dependant oedema: Swelling which due to gravity affects the lowest part of the body. In mobile individuals this will be the ankles, but in bedridden patients this may be the sacrum.

Dextrocardia: Situation when the apex of the heart is in the right chest.

Diabetes: Abnormality of glucose metabolism that is associated with an increased risk of cardiovascular disease.

Diaphragm chestpiece: Part of stethoscope designed to detect high frequency sounds.

Down syndrome: Also known as trisomy 21. Condition in which there is an extra chromosome 21. It is associated with structural cardiac abnormalities, as well as learning difficulties, gut and joint problems.

Dysmorphic: Unusual features, such as single palmar creases, or facial features.

Ejection: Sound caused by the heart ejecting blood in systole. May either be a click from a valve opening, or a murmur from blood passing through the valve.

Finger clubbing: A loss of the normal angle between the nail bed and the skin progressing to a bulbous swelling of the terminal phalanges. This may also affect the toes. It may be congenital, or associated with cardiac, pulmonary, liver or gut disease.

Hypertension: High blood pressure. Definition depends upon age and the context of the measurement.

Intercostal: Between the ribs.

Lipid status: Level of cholesterol and triglycerides in the blood. Abnormally high levels or imbalances may predispose to cardiovascular disease.

Marfan syndrome: Condition due to abnormality of collagen which is characterized by tall stature, hypermobility of the joint, and may involve lens dislocation and cardiac involvement with mitral valve prolapse and aortic root dilatation or rupture.

Myxomatous: Jelly like thickening of a valve.

Obesity: Excess fatty tissue.

Orthopnoea: Breathlessness on lying flat. This may be due to cardiac or pulmonary disease.

Palpitations: An awareness of the heartbeat in the chest.

Paroxysmal nocturnal dyspnoea: Breathlessness which wakens a patient from sleep and is relieved by sitting up. It may be associated with a cough and frothy or lightly blood stained sputum.

Phonocardiogram: A recording of heart sounds.

Pleural effusions: Excess fluid present between the two layers of the pleura.

Regurgitation: Leaking of a valve.

Sphygmomanometer: Device for measuring blood pressure.

Stenosis: Narrowing of a valve.

Stethoscope: Acoustic instrument which allows transmission and amplification of the heart sounds from the chest wall to the listener.

Syncope: Symptom. Sudden loss of conciousness.

Systole: Phase of the cardiac cycle. Usually refers to ventricular systole, but the atrial systole is during the last third of ventricular diastole. When referring to blood pressure, this means the higher reading.

Tachycardia: Fast heart rate. Depends on age (children have faster heart rates than adults). May be sinus, i.e. normal, or due to an arrhythmia, i.e. abnormal.

Valsalva manouvre: Raising intrathoracic and intra-abdominal pressure by exhaling against a closed glottis. Occurs during childbirth, and when straining to defecate.

Vasovagal: Applied to syncope or bradycardia caused by overactivity of the vasovagal nerve.

Xanthomata: Yellow or orange deposits of lipid in the skin. Around the eyes these are known as xanthelasma, and may be normal in the elderly.

Index